YOUR KNOWLEDGE HAS VALUE

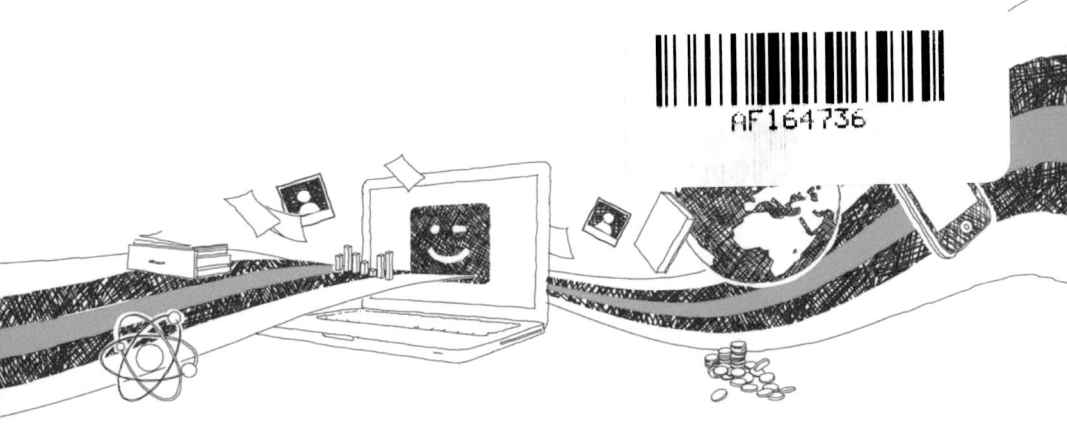

- We will publish your bachelor's and master's thesis, essays and papers

- Your own eBook and book -
  sold worldwide in all relevant shops

- Earn money with each sale

Upload your text at www.GRIN.com
and publish for free

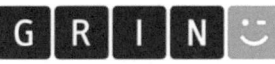

Bibliographic information published by the German National Library:

The German National Library lists this publication in the National Bibliography; detailed bibliographic data are available on the Internet at http://dnb.dnb.de .

This book is copyright material and must not be copied, reproduced, transferred, distributed, leased, licensed or publicly performed or used in any way except as specifically permitted in writing by the publishers, as allowed under the terms and conditions under which it was purchased or as strictly permitted by applicable copyright law. Any unauthorized distribution or use of this text may be a direct infringement of the author s and publisher s rights and those responsible may be liable in law accordingly.

Imprint:

Copyright © 2017 GRIN Verlag, Open Publishing GmbH
Print and binding: Books on Demand GmbH, Norderstedt Germany
ISBN: 9783668504868

This book at GRIN:

http://www.grin.com/en/e-book/371804/the-debate-between-legalizing-marijuana-and-its-benefits-for-medical-purposes

Hassan Nawaz

The Debate between legalizing Marijuana and its Benefits for Medical Purposes. A Pros and Cons Analysis

GRIN Publishing

GRIN - Your knowledge has value

Since its foundation in 1998, GRIN has specialized in publishing academic texts by students, college teachers and other academics as e-book and printed book. The website www.grin.com is an ideal platform for presenting term papers, final papers, scientific essays, dissertations and specialist books.

Visit us on the internet:

http://www.grin.com/

http://www.facebook.com/grincom

http://www.twitter.com/grin_com

The Debate between legalizing Marijuana and its Benefits for Medical Purposes. A Pros and Cons Analysis

Marijuana is also referred to as cannabis. It is among the drugs which alters the perception and the functioning of the human brain. It is obtained from the dried leaves of the hemp plant. Marijuana is occasionally used for medicinal purposes, in which case it is administered in small dosages. However, its use may include such purposes as leisure and recreation, where in such situations it is ingested in large amounts. Marijuana remains an illegal drug in most countries, wherein individuals in possession of its risk subjection to jail service. However, there are a number of countries with a differing opinion and have legalized the drug for individual and general use.

In the environments where it is prohibited, the concerned legal authorities consider the drug as having no medical advantages and only resulting in negative health repercussions to individuals. The debate between the legal validity in the use of marijuana and the benefits realized in the use of the drug for medicinal purposes leads to the conclusion that marijuana has more advantages than disadvantages, when adopted and used in a responsible manner Pope (521).

The use of the marijuana drug and popularity of the same continues to gain audience among young individuals who focus on its use as beneficial to health, rather than harmful. The cannabis plant in indigenous to Asia, but is currently used the world over. The ever increasing numbers among individuals who use the drug has basis on continued protests from the public, on the benefits associated with legalization of the drug. There are several health advantages that are associated with the use of marijuana, which also account significantly, to the widespread use of the drug. Some of the advantages associated with the use of the drug include: treatment of eye dysfunctions – such as Glaucoma, controlling seizures that result from epilepsy, reduction of anxiety, pain reliever – such as in the case of multiple sclerosis, treatment of post-traumatic stress disorder and helping the brain to cope after the event of a stroke.

The occurrence of eye dysfunctions more often than not results in the loss of sight ability. Gieringer, Rosenthal and Carter (99) note that among such eye dysfunctions is glaucoma, which causes gradual deterioration of eye health and steadily leads to complete loss of eyesight. The disease is characteristic of pressure exertion on an individual's eyeballs. The marijuana plant comes in handy in helping ease pain in such a situation. Marijuana further reduces the pressure exerted on the eye as a result of occurrence of glaucoma, and consequently keeps the associated pain at bay (Gieringer, Rosenthal and Carter, 99).

The use of marijuana for the treatment of eye disorders such as the occurrence of glaucoma is possible in the ingestion of the drug in prescribed dosages from qualified medical practitioners. The National eye institute, a notable organization in the treatment of eye disorders, carried out extensive research on the usefulness of using marijuana for the treatment of eye dysfunctions – and specifically, glaucoma. The organization made the conclusion that the drug is efficient in the treatment and control of eye inflammatory diseases. When the drug is ingested in large doses, it is more likely than not to result in failure of relieving such pain as associated with eye disorders.

Further, marijuana is considered useful in the control of seizures that are characteristic of epileptic individuals (Shorvon, Perucca and Engel, 316). Initial experiments intended for validation of the usefulness of marijuana in the prevention of epileptic seizures produced positive results. The results of the experiment proved that marijuana, when taken in appropriate dosages, prevents individuals from falling into seizures within the span of a considerable amount of time. Marijuana has the potential of calming the brain, which enables one maintain a relatively high degree of control over the occurrence of seizures.

Relaxation of the brain muscles is initiated through intake of small quantities of the drug, as administered by professional healthcare providers. However, it is noteworthy that marijuana does not treat or heal epilepsy; it only lessens the intensity associated with the disease's seizures. Hence, a considerable intake of a prescribed dosage of the drug is likely to result in more benefits than harm in the treatment of epileptic seizures. In addition to the effective alleviation of seizures associated with marijuana, it is cost effective. Alternative forms of treatment meant in assisting patients overcome seizures are rather expensive. Patients who experience seizures but are unable to meet the financial demands of expensive medication are able to utilize marijuana, which serves an equally useful function.

Moreover, marijuana has use in the reduction of anxiety in an individual (Stahl, Stephen and Moore, 18). The drug triggers the release of selected chemicals in the body, which provide assistance for achievement of a stable emotional predisposition. The use of marijuana for ease of an individual's anxiety requires careful use. The over-use of the drug is likely to result in the same effects it is assumed to counter. The occurrence of anxiety is associated with the ingestion of large quantities of marijuana, for an individual. It is further possible for individuals to experience uncontrollable feelings of anxiety. In the course of such situations, the individuals involved are able to find assistance through ingestion of small dosages of the drug. The extreme repercussions likely to manifest in users of the drug include paranoid behavior, with focuses on different elements in the environment, as familiar to the world of the patient.

In addition, the use of marijuana is considerably effective for relieving pain in the case that one suffers from pain-characterized diseases such as multiple sclerosis. Sclerosis attack muscle tissues in the body of a patient and induce pain through affliction of the nerve endings. Other numerous drugs are proven not to have the ability of easing the pain associated with such muscle pain (Holland, Murray and Reingold, 4). However, the adoption and use of marijuana gives evidence of reduced pain among users of the same for the specific reasons. The drug presumably numbs the nerve endings that lead to the muscles at pain, hence the brain of the patient is not able to record continued painful experiences. Thus individuals are afforded a relaxed sensation and detachment from a continuous state of pain and physical discomfort.

In consistence with pain relieve in the body, the use of marijuana also relieves patients of the discomfort associated with arthritis. Chemical elements extracted from the marijuana drug aided in relieving patients suffering from rheumatoid arthritis, of their pain. The chemical induces relaxation, which enables the patient focus less on the pain they experience in their bodies.

Moreover, marijuana is considerably effective in the treatment of Post-Traumatic stress Disorder [PTSD]. The disorder is common among war veterans who retire from service. Upon their return home, from war, many of the ex-soldiers remain unable to cope with the environment outside the force. In severe circumstances, individuals experience traumatic effects of their war engagements, long after the war is over. As a coping mechanism against the traumatic effects of retirement from service and adjustment to a new life, the use of marijuana is prescribed in appropriate dosages, as an additional method of enabling the concerned individuals cope with the traumatic experiences (Taylor, 96). The use of marijuana for the treatment of stress and trauma-related experiences is considerably most effective in appropriate dosages. Though the intake of the drug in large amounts ironically yields similar results, it more often than not leads to additional negative health implications on the concerned individual.

Finally, the experience of traumatic events in an individual's life such as stroke, are likely to leave the patients with brain-health instability. The recovery path of a patient's brain condition after such eventualities has basis on the kind of medication administered to the patient. Appropriate doses of the marijuana drug are effective in helping the brain cope with traumatic experiences. The after effects of traumatic events, such as stroke, which have effects on the brain of an individual require an effective form of treatment. The effective form of treatment not only provides an opportunity for future positive-health in the state of the brain, but ensures faster rejuvenation back to a functioning state.

The advantages associated with the use of marijuana for medication purposes, far outweigh the negative consequences associated with its use. Nonetheless, the negative consequences in the use of the drug are notable for lasting negative effects in patients. Arguments that prevail against the use of marijuana, whether for clinical of procreative reasons include: hyperactivity that more often than not leads to addiction to the drug, mental illness and poor health. It is noteworthy that the problems associated with the intake of marijuana occur in cases where the concerned parties consume large amounts of the drug. The inevitable end-results associated with unregulated marijuana intake are consequences on the individuals involved Leonard (07).

The different organization in various countries mandated with research into the properties of drugs and harmful substance categorize marijuana as a harmful drug substance. The major effects associated with drug and substances abuse in an individual includes the alteration of 'normal' function of the body. Arguments presented by Doweiko (416) indicate that drugs and substances categorized as 'harmful' and thus illegal in many countries, alters the perception of an individual towards reality. Marijuana is notable for increasing brain hyperactivity when ingested in large quantities. Such a state of hyperactivity is prolonged over long periods. A users attempt at ensuring the continued state of hyperactivity leads to further usage of the drug, and hence addiction. At the stage of addiction, a marijuana user is unable to function in a stable manner without the intake of the drug on a regular basis Doweiko (416).

Moreover, individuals who have a historical reputation in the use of marijuana are reported to perform lower on intelligence tests, compared to other individuals who are free from the use of the drug. The prolonged use of the drug arguably leads to decreased brain performance and alters the intelligence of an individual (Pertwee, 254). Through an alteration of one's perception of reality, marijuana is likely to lead an individual to make unrealistic and unprecedented life-changing decisions. (Pertwee, 254) further argues that the reduction in intelligence performance of an individual over time, linked to the use of marijuana, has a direct correlation with deterioration in the general health of the concerned person. Reduced body immunity presents the main challenge in the attempt at ensuring healthy bodily pre-dispositions of marijuana users.

The arguments presented against the use of marijuana offer a 'single-sided' perspective on the effects associated with the use of the drug. Marijuana is clinically proven as a constituent of numerous medicinal components, which possess healing properties for different human ailments. However, the different medicinal elements contained in the drug need be ingested in appropriate portions for experience of healing and maintenance of stable health in the case of ailment. Thus, the current medical properties and advantages associated with the use of marijuana are currently not exhaustive, where medical experts continue engagement in analysis and determination of more potential uses of the drug. Further, arguments in favor of abolishment of the drug disregard the fact that negative effects associated with the use of marijuana are due to intake of the drug in large proportions Ogborne (1685).

Marijuana, an extract from the hemp plant, remains one of the most scrutinized drugs in the market over its legality and effectiveness in the provision of treatment. Arguments in favor of using the drug clearly prove that effective medication is possible through the use of marijuana, on condition that it is administered in appropriate dosages by a healthcare provider. On the other hand arguments presented against the popularization of the drug indicate that marijuana retains no health benefits and only serves harm to the involved individuals. It is clear that marijuana has multiple medicinal advantages and value. The realization of benefits associated with the use of the drug is only beneficial within the confines of appropriate knowledge concerning its use.

Extensive studies and research prevails on the potential medicinal uses of marijuana. There exist numerous beneficial properties of the drug arising from past research and application. Failure of gaining efficient knowledge and applicability of marijuana is set to overlook the substantive medicinal application of the drug.

References

Doweiko, Harold E. *Concepts of Chemical Dependency*. Pacific Grove, Calif: Cengage Learning, 2011. Print.

Gieringer, Dale H, Ed Rosenthal, and Gregory T. Carter. *Marijuana Medical Handbook: Practical Guide to the Therapeutic Uses of Marijuana*. Oakland, Calif: Quick American, 2008. Print.

Holland, Nancy J, T J. Murray, and Stephen C. Reingold. *Multiple Sclerosis: A Guide for the Newly Diagnosed*. New York, N.Y: Demos Medical Pub, 2007. Print.

Leonard, B., and National Institute on Drug Abuse. *The Marijuana: Facts for Teens*. Bethesda, Md.: National Institute on Drug Abuse, National Institutes of Health, 2004. Print.

Ogborne, Alan C., Reginald G. Smart, and Edward M. Adlaf. "Self-reported medical use of marijuana: a survey of the general population." *Canadian Medical Association Journal* 162.12 (2000): 1685-1686.

Pertwee, R G. *Handbook of Cannabis*. Oxford: Oxford University Press, 2014. Print.

Pope, Harrison G., and Deborah Yurgelun-Todd. "The residual cognitive effects of heavy marijuana use in college students." *Jama* 275.7 (1996): 521-527.

Shorvon, S D, Emilio Perucca, and Jerome Engel. *The Treatment of Epilepsy*. Chichester, UK: Wiley-Blackwell, 2009. Print.

Stahl, Stephen M, and Bret A. Moore. *Anxiety Disorders: A Guide for Integrating Psychopharmacology and Psychotherapy*. , 2013. Print.

Taylor, Steven. *Advances in the Treatment of Posttraumatic Stress Disorder: Cognitive-behavioral Perspectives*. New York: Springer Pub. Co, 2004. print.

YOUR KNOWLEDGE HAS VALUE

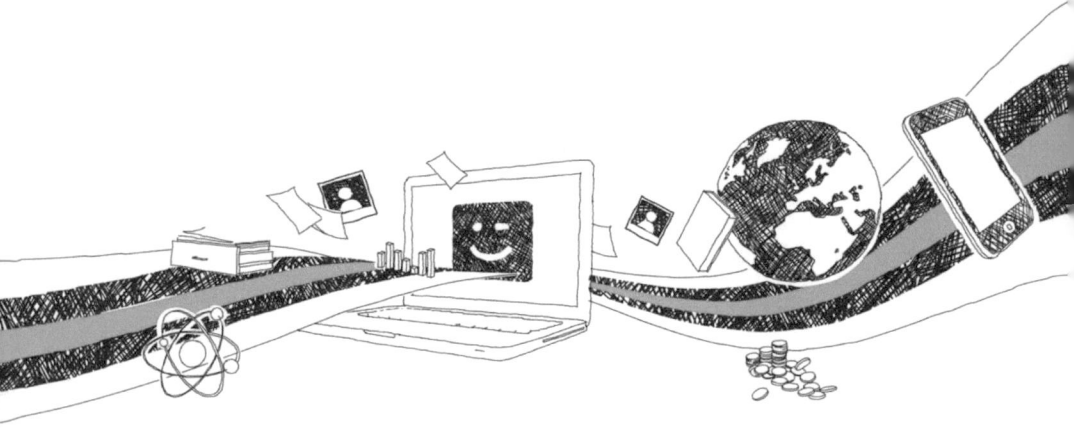

- We will publish your bachelor's and master's thesis, essays and papers

- Your own eBook and book - sold worldwide in all relevant shops

- Earn money with each sale

Upload your text at www.GRIN.com and publish for free